Contents

Preface	2
Reception	5
Anamnesis	11
Massage	23
Manual therapy	28
PNF	38
Mulligan	44
Exercises	47
Gait training	55
Lymphatic drainage	57
Electrotherapy	61
Pelvic floor exercises	64
Breathing therapy	68
Useful	71
Thanks	73
Bibliography	74

Preface

Who am I?

My name is Caroline Braun and I created the Little Physio.
I studied translation and worked as a freelance translator.
I then decided to change my way of living and became a physiotherapist / physical therapist.
I've been working as a physical therapist for over 10 years in different hospitals as well as in private practices.

Why did I create Little Physio?

My experience has shown me the difficulties of treating patients who don't speak the same language.
It's difficult and even sometimes impossible to diagnose or treat the patient correctly.
The consequences for the patient are disastrous.

Many people think that the patient has to speak the language of the country he or she lives in.
Even if correct it's also not always possible.
Some people are not able to learn or have just arrived.
Others might be on vacation or are only here temporarily to work.

I am a physical therapist and my job is not to judge but to treat the patients.
And I have to treat them the best I can.

That's why I created "Little Physio".

This translator enables the therapist to communicate and to treat foreign patients.

Your therapy will become easier and better.

The book is divided into 14 chapters like "Reception", "Massage", "Manual therapy", "Exercises" and so on. This makes it easier and faster for you to find the sentences you need.

In addition to the book, you have the opportunity to get the **Little Physio App for mobile phones and tabs, iphone and ipad.**

The Apps are available on the Apple Appstore and on the Googleplaystore.

The **Little Physio Apps are the audio version of the books**.

It is as easy as clicking on the needed sentence and your cell phone or tab "speaks" it out in the foreign language.

You can see a demo on:

littlephysio.com

or on

youtube

I became a physical therapist to help others, no matter if they speak my language or not.

Now, it is possible!

Reception

Réception

1. Hello
Bonjour

2. My name is
Je suis...

3. Do you have a doctor's prescription?
Avez-vous une ordonnance?

4. Yes
Oui

5. No
Non

6. Do you have your insurance card?
Avez-vous une carte vitale?

7. Would you please bring the insurance card next time?

Pouvez-vous apporter votre carte vitale la prochaine fois?

8. Would you please write down your phone number?

Pouvez-vous m'écrire votre numéro de téléphone, s'il vous plait?

9. There is a mistake in the prescription. You have to go back to your doctor and have him issue a new one.

Il y a une erreur sur l'ordonnance, vous devez retourner chez le medecin pour qu'il la corrige.

10. Do you have a report / X-ray / CT- images from your doctor?

Avez-vous un rapport du médecin / des radios, des tomographies?

11. Would you please bring the x-rays / the report with you next time?

Pouvez-vous amener les radios, les tomographies la prochaine fois?

12. Here are your appointments
Voici vos rendez-vous

13. If these appointments don't work for you, please let me know.
Si les rendez-vous ne vous conviennent pas, dites le moi

14. This one doesn't work?
Ça ne va pas?

15. Not on this day at all?
Pas ce jour là?

16. Rather in the morning?
Plutôt le matin

17. Rather in the afternoon?
Plutôt l'après-midi

18. Monday
Lundi

19. Tuesday
Mardi

20. Wednesday
Mercredi

21. Thursday
Jeudi

22. Friday
Vendredi

23. Saturday
Samedi

24. Sunday
Dimanche

25. I'm sorry, you are too early
Je suis désolée, vous êtes en avance

26. I'm sorry, you are too late
Je suis désolée, vous êtes en retard

27. This week won't work
   Ce n'est pas possible cette semaine

28. Today doesn't work
   Ce n'est pas possible aujourd´hui

29. Not before next week
   A partir de la semaine prochaine

30. Not before next month
   A partir du mois prochain

31. The therapist is on vacation
   La / le thérapeute est en vacances

32. The therapist is ill
   La / le thérapeute est malade

33. Would you like to work with a different therapist?
   Voulez-vous un autre thérapeute ?

34. Yes
   Oui

35. No

Non

36. Would you like to continue with the same therapist?

Voulez-vous avoir le / la même thérapeute ?

37. Would you rather wait until your therapist is back?

Voulez-vous attendre que le / la thérapeute revienne ?

38. Here is your bill.

Voici votre facture.

39. Would you like to pay now?

Voulez-vous payer maintenant ?

40. Do you want to pay cash?

Voulez-vous payer contant ?

Anamnesis

Anamnese

1. Please undress
   Deshabillez vous s´il vous plait

2. Can you please take off your top ?
   Pouvez-vous enlevez votre haut?

3. Can you please take off your pants?
   Pouvez-vous enlever votre pantalon?

4. Can you please take off your skirt?
   Pouvez-vous enlever votre jupe?

5. Are you in pain?
   Avez-vous des douleurs?

6. Yes
   Oui

7. No

Non .

8. Show me where it hurts

Montrez moi où vous avez des douleurs

9. Where does it hurt?

Où sont vos douleurs ?

10. Is the pain radiating into your arm?

Les douleurs se diffusent-elles dans le bras?

11. Is the pain radiating into your leg?

Les douleurs se diffusent-elles dans la jambe?

12. Where does the pain radiate into?

Où les douleurs se diffusent-elles ?

13. Show me

Montrez moi

14. Do you feel numbness?

Avez vous des zones insensibles?

15. Where?

Où?

16. Do you have paralytic symptoms?

Avez-vous des paralysies, faiblesses musculaires?

17. Do you feel formication?

Avez-vous des fourmis?

18. Where?

Où?

19. When did it start?

Depuis quand?

20. For days

Depuis plusieurs jours

21. For weeks
Depuis plusieurs semaines

22. For months
Depuis plusieurs mois

23. For years
Depuis plusieurs années

24. What does the pain feel like?
Comment est la douleur?

25. Acute
Lancinante

26. Dull
Diffuse

27. Dragging
Par élancements

28. Did the pain develop slowly?

La douleur a-t-elle commencé doucement?

29. Did the pain develop fast?

La douleur a-t-elle commencé d´un seul coup?

30. Does the pain last for a long time?

La douleur persiste-t-elle longtemps?

31. Several seconds

Plusieurs secondes

32. Several minutes

Plusieurs minutes

33. Several hours

Plusieurs heures

34. Several days

Plusieurs jours

35. Did you have an accident?
Avez-vous eu un accident?

36. Have you had treatment yet?
Avez-vous déjà recu des soins ?

37. Yes
Oui

38. No
Non

39. Do you have high blood pressure?
Faites-vous de l´hypertension?

40. Do you have diabetes?
Avez-vous le diabète?

41. Are you dizzy?
Avez-vous des vertiges?

42. Are you pregnant?
Etes-vous enceinte?

43. What month?
Depuis combien de mois?

44. Do you take pain killers?
Prenez vous des antidouleurs?

45. Do you take blood thinning medication?
Prenez vous des anticoagulants? / des médicaments?

46. Do you have problems with your thyroid?
Avez-vous des problèmes de thyroide?

47. Do you have heart problems?
Avez-vous des problèmes cardiaques?

48. Do you have a headache?
Avez-vous des maux de tête?

49. Did you have surgery?

Vous êtes vous fait opérer?

50. When did you have surgery?

Quand vous êtes vous fait opérer?

51. A few days ago

Il y a quelques jours

52. A few months ago

Il y a quelques mois

53. A few years ago

Il y a quelques années

54. You have to see a doctor.

Vous devez aller chez le médecin

55. Does it hurt when you are moving?

Avez-vous des douleurs liées à une activité / pendant une activité?

56. Do you have pain while resting?

Avez-vous des douleurs au repos?

57. When does it hurt most? When is the pain worst?

Quand les douleurs sont-elles maximales?

58. In the morning

Le matin

59. In the evening

Le soir

60. At night

La nuit

61. Always the same

Toujours pareil

62. While going up

En marchant quand ça monte

63. While going down

En marchant quand ça descend

64. Going up the stairs

En montant les escaliers

65. Going down the stairs

En descendant les escaliers

66. While sitting for a long time

Quand vous restez assis(e) longtemps?

67. After sitting for a long time

Après être resté assis(s) longtemps?

68. While doing small movements?

Lors de très petits mouvements?

69. Were you in the hospital / in rehab?

Êtes-vous allé(e) à l'hôpital/ en cure?

70. For how long?
  Combien de temps?

71. Several days
  Plusieurs jours

72. Several weeks
  Plusieurs semaines

73. Several months
  Plusieurs mois

74. When did you get discharged from the hospital?
  Quand êtes-vous sorti(e) de l'hôpital ?

75. Yesterday
  Hier

76. The day before yesterday
  Avant-hier

77. A few days ago

　Il y a quelques jours

78. How many?

　Combien ?

79. A few weeks ago

　Il y a quelques semaines

80. A few months ago

　Il y a quelques mois

Massage

Massage

1. Please get undressed

Vous pouvez vous déshabiller

2. Can you please take off your top?

Pouvez vous enlever votre haut?

3. Can you please take off your pants?

Pouvez vous enlever votre pantalon?

4. Can you please take off your skirt?

Pouvez vous enlever votre jupe?

5. Lie down on your back

Couchez vous sur le dos

6. Lie down on your stomach

Couchez vous sur le ventre

7. Lie down on your right side
Couchez vous sur le côté droit

8. Lie down on your left side
Couchez vous sur le côté gauche

9. This is for your head
La tête ici, s´il vous plait

10. Would you like a blanket?
Voulez-vous une couverture?

11. Are you cold?
Avez-vous froid

12. Are you too warm?
Avez-vous trop chaud?

13. Put your right arm down
Mettez votre bras drois en bas

14. Put your right arm next to your head

Mettez votre bras drois en haut

15. Align your right arm alongside your body

Mettez votre bras droit le long du corps

16. Put your left arm down

Mettez votre bras gauche en bas

17. Put your left arm next to your head

Mettez votre bras gauche en haut

18. Align your left arm alongside your body

Mettez votre bras gauche le long du corps

19. Sit down please.

Asseyez-vous, s´il vous plait

20. Relax your shoulders

Détendez vos épaules

21. Please look straigt ahead

Regardez devant vous

22. Does it hurt?

Ça fait mal?

23. Do I hurt you?

Est-ce que je vous fais mal?

24. Show me where it hurts.

Montrez moi ou ça fait mal

25. Is the pressure ok?

Est-ce-que la pression est bonne / est-ce que j'appuie bien?

26. Yes?

Oui ?

27. No?

Non?

28. Harder?

Plus fort ?

29. Softer?

Moins fort?

30. Better?

C'est mieux?

31. Worse?

C'est moins bien?

Manual therapy

Thérapie manuelle

1. Please get undressed

Vous pouvez vous déshabiller

2. Can you please take off your top?

Pouvez vous enlever votre haut?

3. Can you please take off your pants?

Pouvez vous enlever votre pantalon?

4. Can you please take off your skirt?

Pouvez vous enlever votre jupe?

5. Where does it hurt?

Oú avez-vous mal / des douleurs?

6. Has it improved since the last treatment?

Est-ce que vous allez mieux depuis la dernière thérapie?

7. Has it gotten worse?
Est-ce moins bien qu'avant?

8. Has the pain increased?
Avez-vous plus de douleurs maintenant?

9. Has the pain gotten less?
Avez-vous moins de douleurs maintenant?

10. Where does it hurt now?
Où sont les douleurs maintenant / où avez-vous mal maintenant

11. Stand on one leg please.
Tenez vous sur une jambe

12. Please stand on the other leg now.
Maintenant, tenez vous sur l'autre jambe

13. Stand on your heels
Tenez vous debout seulement sur les talons

14. Stand on your tiptoes
Tenez vous debout sur la pointes des pieds

15. Sit down please

Asseyez-vous

16. Round your back

Faites le dos rond

17. Put your chin to your chest

Mettez la tête en avant / posez le menton sur votre sternum

18. Does it pull?

Ça tire?

19. Is it painful?

Ça fait mal / c´est douloureux?

20. Is the pain less now?

C´est moins douloureux comme ça?

21. Is the pain worse now?

C´est plus douloureux comme ça?

22. Better?

C´est mieux ?

23. Worse?
C'est pire?

24. Put your head back
Soulevez la tête

25. Lift your head up, look up
Regardez en l'air

26. Put your head down, look down
Regardez vers le bas / baissez la tête

27. Turn your head to the left
Tournez la tête à gauche

28. Turn your head to the right
Tournez la tête à droite

29. Tilt your head to the left
Penchez la tête à gauche

30. Tilt your head to the right
Penchez la tête à droite

31. Relax
Détendez / restez détendu(e)

32. Do not help. I will do the movements, you relax
N´essayez pas de m'aider, je fais le mouvement, vous restez détendu(e)

33. Put your arms up
Levez les bras

34. Put your right arm up
Levez le bras droit

35. Put your right arm down
Baissez le bras droit

36. Put your left arm up
Levez le bras gauche

37. Put your left arm down
Baissez le bras gauche

38. Bend your leg
Pliez la jambe

39. Extend your leg
   Tendez la jambe

40. Bend your knee
   Pliez le genou

41. Extend your knee
   Tendez le genou

42. Lift your leg
   Levez la jambe

43. Lie on your back
   Couchez vous sur le dos

44. Lie on your stomach
   Couchez vous sur le ventre

45. Lie on your right side
   Couchez vous sur le côté droit

46. Lie on your left side
   Couchez vous sur le côté gauche

47. Put your head here, please
La tête ici, s´il vous plait

48. Sit down
Asseyez vous

49. Please participate with ease
Faites le mouvement avec moi.

50. Press against my resistance
Poussez contre ma pression

51. Press harder
Poussez plus fort

52. Press not so hard
Poussez moins fort

53. This is an exercise to do at home
Ceci est un exercice à faire à la maison

54. Bend your legs and pull your knees to your thighs
Pliez les jambes et posez les pieds sous les genoux

55. Tighten your Abdomen
Contractez les muscles du ventre / faites marcher vos abdominaux

56. Squeeze your buttocks
Contractez les muscles fessiers

57. Tense your legs
Contractez les muscles des jambes

58. Tense your arms
Contractez les muscles des bras

59. Relax
Détendez vous / vos muscles

60. It might hurt a little
Il est possible que ça fasse un peu mal

61. I will show you first, then you repeat
Je vous montre, ensuite vous le faites

62. Do 3 sets with 10 repetitions
Faites trois séries à 10 répétitions

63. Do 3 sets with 15 repetitions
Faites trois séries à 15 répétitions

64. Do 3 sets with 20 repetitions
Faites trois séries à 20 répétitions

65. Do 3 sets with 30 repetitions
Faites trois séries à 30 répétitions

66. Once a week
Une fois par semaine

67. Twice a week
Deux fois par semaine

68. Three times a week
Trois fois par semaine

69. Once a day
Une fois par jour

70. Twice a day
Deux fois par jour

71. Three times a day

Trois fois par jour

72. Do the exercise in front of a mirror

Faites l´exercice devant le miroir

73. Sit down in front of a mirror

Asseyez vous devant le miroir

74. Stand in front of a mirror

Restez debout devant le miroir

75. It is not supposed to hurt

Ça ne doit pas faire mal

76. This is not supposed to happen

Ça ne doit pas arriver

PNF

Facilitation neuromusculaire par la proprioception

1. Lie on your back
   Couchez vous sur le dos

2. Lie on your stomach
   Couchez vous sur le ventre

3. Lie on your right side
   Couchez vous sur le côté droit

4. Lie on your left side
   Couchez vous sur le côté gauche

5. Put your head here, please
   La tête ici, s´il vous plait

6. I will show you what the movement should look like
Je vous montre comment faire le mouvement.

7. I will do the movement, relax your arm
Je fais le mouvement, vous laissez le bras détendu

8. I will do the movement, relax your leg
Je fais le mouvement, vous laissez la jambe détendue

9. Press against my resistance now
Maintenant, appuyez/poussez contre ma pression

10. Open your hand and extend your fingers
Ouvrez les doigts et la main

11. Close your hand aroung mine
Fermez les doigts et la main

12. Extend your arm
Tendez le coude

13. Bend your elbow
   Pliez le coude

14. Put your leg up
   Levez la jambe

15. Put your leg down
   Baissez la jambe

16. Tense your leg in this direction
   Contractez la jambe dans cette direction

17. Bend your knee
   Pliez le genou

18. Extend your knee
   Tendez le genou

19. Bend your hips
   Pliez la hanche

20. Extend your hips
Tendez la hanche

21. Relax
Détendez vous / détendez vos muscles

22. More
Plus

23. Less
Moins

24. Harder
Plus fort

25. Softer
Moins fort

26. Slower
Moins vite

27. Faster
Plus vite

28. Press upward
Appuyez, poussez vers le haut

29. Press downward
Appuyez, poussez vers le bas

30. Now in the other direction
Maintenant dans l'autre direction

31. Towards your opposite shoulder
En direction de l'épaule de l'autre côté

32. Towards your opposite hip
En direction de la hanche de l´autre côté

33. Towards the ear
Vers l´oreille

34. Towards the nose
Vers le nez

35. Towards the window
Vers la fenêtre

36. Towards the door
Vers la porte

37. Towards the wall
Vers le mur

38. Towards the clock
Vers l'horloge

Mulligan

Mulligan

1. Show me which movement causes the pain

Montrez moi quel mouvement vous provoque des douleurs

2. Relax

Détendez vous / restez détendu

3. Repeat the movement once more

Maintenant, recommencez le mouvement.

4. Is it better?

C´est mieux?

5. Do you have pain going upstairs?

Avez vous des douleurs en montant les escaliers?

6. Do you have pain going downstairs?

Avez vous des douleurs en descandant les escaliers?

7. Is it better like this?

C'est mieux comme ça?

8. You are not supposed to be in pain. Please say Stop if it hurts

Vous ne devez pas avoir de douleurs, si ça fait mal, dites stop.

9. If the strap hurts, I can put a pad between you and the strap

Si la ceinture vous fait mal, je peux mettre un petit coussin entre vous et la ceinture.

10. You can do this exercise with a towel at home

Vous pouvez faire cet exercice à la maison avec une serviette.

11. you can do this exercise at home with an elastic band

Vous pouvez faire cet exercice à la maison avec une bande élastique.

12. You can do this exercise at home with a stick

Vous pouvez faire cet exercice à la maison avec un baton.

13. The ball can be purchased at a sporting goods store

Vous pouvez acheter la balle dans un magasin de sport.

14. The elastic band can be purchased at a sporting goods store

Vous pouvez acheter la bande élastique dans un magasin de sport.

15. It should be red

Elle doit être rouge

16. It should be green

Elle doit être verte.

Exercises

Exercices

1. Bend
Pliez

2. Extend
Tendez

3. Flex
Contractez vos muscles

4. Relax
Détendez vos muscles

5. Move your buttocks backwards
Le postérieur en arrière

6. tense your abdomen / do not relax
Contractez vos abdominaux / gardez les abdominaux contractés

7. Remain like this for a few seconds, then relax

Restez comme ça quelques secondes, ensuite détendez vos muscles

8. Do not move

Il ne doit y avoir aucun mouvement.

9. This is for your coordination

Ceci est pour la coordination

10. Do 3 sets with 10 repetitions

Faites trois séries à 10 répétitions

11. Do 3 sets with 15 repetitions

Faites trois séries à 15 répétitions

12. Do 3 sets with 20 repetitions

Faites trois séries à 20 répétitions

13. Do 3 sets with 30 repetitions

Faites trois séries à 30 répétitions

14. Take a break between the sets
Faites une pause entre les séries

15. A few seconds
Quelques secondes

16. A few minutes
Quelques minutes

17. How many
Combien

18. Once a week
Une fois par semaine

19. Twice a week
Deux fois par semaine

20. Three times a week
Trois fois par semaine

21. Once a day
   Une fois par jour

22. Twice a day
   Deux fois par jour

23. Three times a day
   Trois fois par jour

24. Do the exercise while standing in front of a mirror
   Faites l'exercice devant le miroir

25. Sit in front of the mirror
   Asseyez vous devant le miroir

26. Stand in front of the mirror
   Restez debout devant le miroir

27. This is for strengthening
   Ceci est pour la musculation

28. Do it at home every day
Faites le tous les jours à la maison

29. Do the exercises in front of the mirror so that you can correct yourself
Faites les exercices devant le miroir pour pouvoir corriger les erreurs.

30. This is not supposed to happen
Cela ne doit pas arriver

31. This is wrong
Comme ça, c´est faux

32. This is correct
Comme ça, c´est bien

33. Slow
Lentement

34. Slower
Plus lentement

35. Fast
vite

36. Faster
plus vite

37. don't jerk
Pas de mouvements brusques

38. Your are not supposed to be in pain during the exercise
Vous ne devez pas avoir de douleurs pendant des exercices.

39. If you are in pain doing the exercise please stop and tell me next time you are here.
Si vous avez des douleurs pendant les exercices, ne les faites plus et dites le moi la prochaine fois

40. Did you do the exercises?
Avez-vous fait les exercices?

41. Did you feel any pain?

Avez-vous eu des douleurs?

42. Show me where it hurt?

Montrez moi où vous avez eu des douleurs

43. Show me how you do the exercises?

Montrez moi comment vous faites l'exercice.

44. Stand on your right leg

Tenez vous debout sur la jambe droite

45. Stand on your left leg

Tenez vous debout sur la jambe gauche

46. Stand on one leg

Tenez vous debout sur une jambe

47. This is for balance

Ceci est pour l'équilibre

48. Try not to move

Essayez de ne pas tanguer

49. Try to include this exercise in your daily routine

Essayez d´intégrer ce mouvement dans votre quotidien

Gait training

Reprise de la marche

1. Stand straight
   Tenez vous droit(e)

2. Take smaller steps
   Faites des pas plus petits

3. Take bigger steps
   Faites des pas plus grands

4. Take regular steps
   Faites des pas réguliers

5. Roll your foot from heel to toe
   Roulez bien le pied

6. First on your heel, roll your foot, then press your foot forward to your toes

D´abord le talon, ensuite le pied roule et se propulse en avant avec la pointe du pied

7. The crutch goes on the same side as your injured leg

Les béquilles accompagnent toujours la jambe malade

8. Swing your arms loosely by your body

Laissez les bras détendus le long du corps

Lymphatic drainage

Drainage lymphatique

1. The blood pressure cannot be taken on this arm nor can blood be drawn

On ne doit pas vous faire de prise de sang ou prendre votre tension à ce bras.

2. Preferably you should not get hurt

Vous devez faire attention à ne pas vous blesser

3. You are not allowed to take a hot bath or lie in the sun for too long

Vous ne devez pas prendre de bain brûlant ou prendre de bain de soleil

4. If you have a painful rash, see a doctor immediately

Si vous remarquez une éruption cutanée, rendez vous immédiatement chez le médecin.

5. Put your legs up multiple times per day

Surélevez les jambes souvent, plusieurs fois par jour.

6. Put your leg up several times a day

Surélevez la jambe souvent, plusieurs fois par jour.

7. Put your arm up multiple times a day

Surélevez le bras souvent, plusieurs fois par jour.

8. Do you have a surgical stocking?

Avez-vous un bas de compression?

9. Do you have surgical stockings?

Avez-vous des bas de compression?

10. You have to wear the stocking every day

Vous devez porter le bas tous les jours.

11. You have to wear the stockings every day

Vous devez porter les bas tous les jours.

12. You have to wear the stocking night and day

Vous devez porter le bas jour et nuit.

13. You have to wear the stockings night and day

Vous devez porter les bas jour et nuit.

14. You shouldn't wear tight-fitting clothes
Vous ne devez pas porter de vêtements trop serrés.

15. Lie on your back
Couchez vous sur le dos

16. Lie on your stomach
Tournez vous sur le ventre

17. Can you lie on your stomach or would your rather sit?
Pouvez-vous vous coucher sur le ventre ou préfèrez vous vous assoir?

18. Sit?
Assis(e) ?

19. Put one leg up
Pliez la jambe et posez le pied sous le genoux

20. Put both legs up
Pliez les jambes et posez les pieds sous les genoux

21. Slide a little towards me

Rapprochez vous un peu de moi

22. Slide to the left

Mettez vous un peu plus à gauche

23. Slide to the right

Mettez vous un peu plus à droite

24. Slide up

Mettez vous un peu plus haut

25. Slide down

Mettez vous un peu plus bas

26. Does it hurt?

Ça fait mal?

27. It shouldn't hurt

Ça ne doit pas faire mal

Electrotherapy

Electrothérapie

1. I will attach 2 electrodes

Je vais poser deux électrodes

2. I will attach 4 electrodes

Je vais poser quatre électrodes

3. There is no electricity yet

Il n´y a pas encore de courant électrique

4. I will increase the electricity slowly

Je monte un peu la puissance électrique

5. Tell me, as soon as you feel the electricity

Dites le moi, dès que vous sentez l´électricité

6. Do you feel the electricity?

Sentez-vous l´électricité?

7. It should be comfortable

Ça doit être agréable

8. Is it comfortable?

Est-ce agréable?

9. You should feel the electricity only slightly

Vous ne devez sentir qu'un léger courant électrique

10. I will turn down the electricity until you can't feel it anymore

Je baisse maintenant la puissance électrique jusqu'à ce que vous ne sentiez plus le courant.

11. It will take about 10 minutes

Cela va durer environ dix minutes

12. It will take about 15 minutes

Cela va durer environ quinze minutes

13. It will take about 20 minutes

Cela va durer environ vingt minutes

14. I will take off the electrodes once it is finished

Lorsque c´est terminé, je reviens enlever les électrodes.

15. If you have a problem, call me

S´il y a un problème, appelez moi.

16. I will be next-door

Je suis à côté

Pelvic floor exercises

Rééducation du périnée

short

1. The pelvic floor is the muscle between your pubic bone and your tailbone

Le périnée est un muscle qui se situe entre le pubis et le coccys.

2. Its function is mainly to close the openings there

Sa fonction principale est de fermer les ouvertures qui s´y trouvent.

3. It works together with you abdominal muscles and your diaphragm

Il travaille avec les muscles abdominaux et le diaphragme.

4. In order to strengthen your pelvic floor you have to use these muscles as well

C´est pour cela que ces muscles doivent aussi travailler pour remuscler le périnée.

5. **Try to tense your pelvic floor, acting like have to use the bathroom but you can't go**

    Essayez de contracter le périnée en faisant comme si vous deviez aller aux toilettes mais que vous ne pouviez pas.

Long

1. **The pelvic floor is the muscle between ischial tuberosities, pubic and tailbone**

    Le Périnée est le muscle situé entre les os coxaux latéraux (les os sur lesquels on s´assoit) le coccyx et le pubis.

2. **The pelvic floor helps to control the function of urinating and bowel movement. With regular training you can prevent incontinence or lessen exiting problems**

    La fonction principale du périnée est le contrôle de la continence. Grâce à un entrainement régulier, vous pourrez éviter une incontinence ou améliorer la situation dans le cas d´une incontinence déjà présente.

3. In addition, the pelvic floor holds and supports the organs in your abdomen. That's why regular pelvic floor training works against prolapse problems

Le périnée protège et soutient les organes situés dans le bassin. C'est pour cette raison qu'un entrainement du périnée permet d'éviter une descente d'organes.

4. To fulfill these functions, the pelvic floor works with the abdominal muscles and the diaphragm, which is the most important respiratory muscle.

Afin de fonctionner correctement, le périnée travaille avec les muscles abdominaux et le diaphragme, le muscle respiratoire le plus important.

5. In order to strengthen your pelvic floor you have to use these muscles as well

C'est pour cette raison qu'il faut faire travailler ces muscles afin de remuscler le périnée.

6. Try to tighten your pelvic floor, imagining closing your vagina and anus

Essayez de contracter votre périnée en vous imaginant que vous fermer votre anus et votre vagin.

7. **Try to tighten your pelvic floor, acting like have to use the toilet but you can't go**

   Essayez de contracter votre périnéé en le contractant comme si vous aviez besoin d´aller aux toilettes mais que vous ne pouviez pas.

8. **Inhale deeply. Exhale slowly tensing your abdominal muscles**

   Inspirez profondément, contractez votre ventre et expirez en même temps.

9. **I will show you, and then you do it**

   Je vous montre et ensuite vous le faites.

Breathing therapy

Thérapie respiratoire

1. Inhale through your nose

Inspirez par le nez

2. Exhale through your mouth

Expirez par la bouche

3. I will show you, and then you do it

Je vous montre, ensuite vous le faites.

4. Slowly

Lentement

5. Slower

Plus lentement

6. Fast

Vite

7. Faster
Plus vite

8. Deeply
Profondément

9. Deeper
Plus profondément

10. Casual
Superficiellement

11. More casually
Moins profondément

12. Inhale more into your abdomen
Respirez plus dans le ventre

13. Your abdomen should expand when inhaling
Le ventre doit devenir plus gros lorsque vous inspirez

14. Put your hands on your abdomen

Posez vos mains sur le ventre

15. Put your hands on your ribcage

Posez vos mains sur la cage thoracique

16. Your hands should be moving on your abdomen when inhaling

Votre ventre doit faire bouger vos mains lorsque vous inspirez

Useful

Pratique

1. Hello
Bonjour

2. Goodbye
Au revoir

3. Please
S´il vous plaît

4. Thank you
Merci

5. Relax
Restez relaxé

6. Does it hurt?
C'est douloureux?

7. Is it better now?
C'est mieux comme cela?

8. Harder?
Plus fort?

9. Yes
Oui

10. No
Non

11. I'm sorry, I can't understand you
Je suis désolé, je ne comprends pas

Thanks

I would like to thank all those who helped me to create the Little Physio book and application.

Thanks to the translators and the proof-readers, thanks to my family and my friends who have all participated in this adventure.

Thanks to those who helped with their voice on the apps and the videos.

Special thanks to my husband who programmed the apps for android and apple and for everything else too... :)

Thank you, dear reader for having bought this book or any of my other books.

If you have enjoyed Little Physio,
please leave comments on Amazon.

I would appreciate it very much :)

Bibliography

- **Little Physio** from English into Spanish
- **Little Physio** from English into Italian
- **Little Physio** from English into French
- **Little Physio** from English into German
- **Little Physio** from English into Turkish

and

- **Big Little Physio** from English into Spanish, Italian, French, German and Turkish

www.ingramcontent.com/pod-product-compliance
Lightning Source LLC
Chambersburg PA
CBHW071800170526
45167CB00003B/1114